MY FOOD DIARY
& WORKOUT TRACKER

12 WEEK PLANNER

- This planner belongs to -

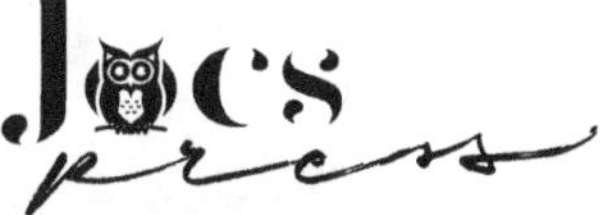

THE ONLY BAD WORKOUT IS THE ONE THAT DIDN'T HAPPEN

Put pen to paper to plan for success, record your stats, track progress + reach your goals!

Our planner is designed to cover your daily exercise and food logs for 12 weeks.

Don't wait until the New Year to set health and fitness goals for yourself. Writing down your workouts each day—doing it in a notebook the old-fashioned way—is an easy way to help keep yourself accountable and help you stay on track.

WEIGHT TRACKER

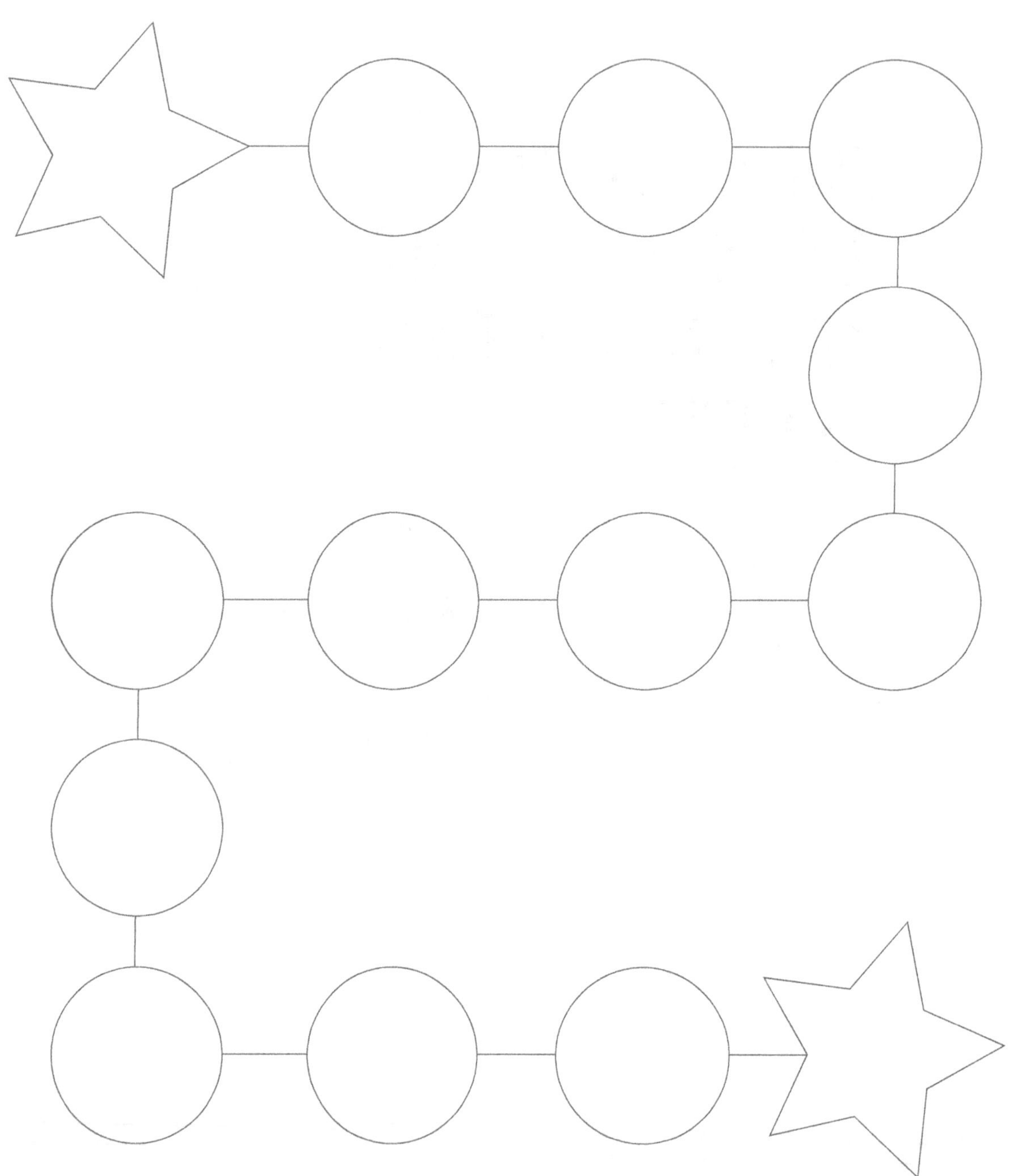

MY 12 WEEK PROGRESS

	WEEK 1	WEEK 2	WEEK 3	WEEK 4	WEEK 5	WEEK 6	WEEK 7
NECK							
UPPER ARM							
CHEST							
WAIST							
HIPS							
UPPER THIGH							
CALF							

	WEEK 8	WEEK 9	WEEK 10	WEEK 11	WEEK 12	INCHES −/+
NECK						
UPPER ARM						
CHEST						
WAIST						
HIPS						
UPPER THIGH						
CALF						

TOTAL DIFFERENCE =

MY DAY

DATE: ___/___/___   M T W T F S S

FOOD JOURNAL

Breakfast

PROTEIN	FATS	CARBS	CALORIES

Lunch

PROTEIN	FATS	CARBS	CALORIES

Dinner

PROTEIN	FATS	CARBS	CALORIES

Snacks

PROTEIN	FATS	CARBS	CALORIES

WATER

○ ○ ○ ○ ○ ○ ○ ○

SLEEP (HRS)

DAILY STEPS

FOCUS

☐ Legs   ☐ Arms   ☐ Abs   ☐ Full body

STRENGTH

EXERCISE	SETS	REPS	WEIGHT

CARDIO

	TIME	DISTANCE	INTENSITY

REST DAY

MY DAY

DATE: _______________ / _______ M T W T F S S

FOOD JOURNAL

Breakfast

PROTEIN	FATS	CARBS	CALORIES

Lunch

PROTEIN	FATS	CARBS	CALORIES

Dinner

PROTEIN	FATS	CARBS	CALORIES

Snacks

PROTEIN	FATS	CARBS	CALORIES

WATER ◯ ◯ ◯ ◯ ◯ ◯ ◯ ◯

SLEEP (HRS)

DAILY STEPS

FOCUS

☐ Legs ☐ Arms ☐ Abs ☐ Full body

STRENGTH

EXERCISE	SETS	REPS	WEIGHT

CARDIO

	TIME	DISTANCE	INTENSITY

REST DAY

MY DAY

DATE: / /   M T W T F S S

FOOD JOURNAL

Breakfast

PROTEIN	FATS	CARBS	CALORIES

Lunch

PROTEIN	FATS	CARBS	CALORIES

Dinner

PROTEIN	FATS	CARBS	CALORIES

Snacks

PROTEIN	FATS	CARBS	CALORIES

WATER

○ ○ ○ ○ ○ ○ ○ ○

SLEEP (HRS)

DAILY STEPS

FOCUS

☐ Legs	☐ Arms	☐ Abs	☐ Full body

STRENGTH

EXERCISE	SETS	REPS	WEIGHT

CARDIO

	TIME	DISTANCE	INTENSITY

REST DAY

MY DAY

DATE: / /

M T W T F S S

FOOD JOURNAL

Breakfast

PROTEIN	FATS	CARBS	CALORIES

Lunch

PROTEIN	FATS	CARBS	CALORIES

Dinner

PROTEIN	FATS	CARBS	CALORIES

Snacks

PROTEIN	FATS	CARBS	CALORIES

WATER

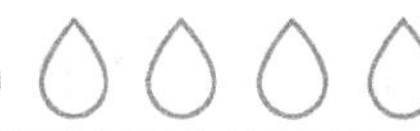

SLEEP (HRS)

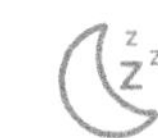

DAILY STEPS

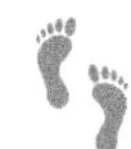

FOCUS

☐ Legs   ☐ Arms   ☐ Abs   ☐ Full body

STRENGTH

EXERCISE	SETS	REPS	WEIGHT

CARDIO

	TIME	DISTANCE	INTENSITY

REST DAY

MY DAY

DATE: / /   M T W T F S S

FOOD JOURNAL

Breakfast

PROTEIN	FATS	CARBS	CALORIES

Lunch

PROTEIN	FATS	CARBS	CALORIES

Dinner

PROTEIN	FATS	CARBS	CALORIES

Snacks

PROTEIN	FATS	CARBS	CALORIES

WATER

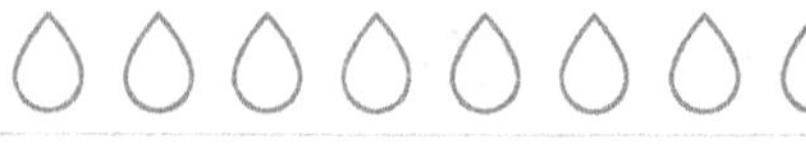

SLEEP (HRS)

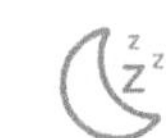

DAILY STEPS

FOCUS

☐ Legs ☐ Arms ☐ Abs ☐ Full body

STRENGTH

EXERCISE	SETS	REPS	WEIGHT

CARDIO

	TIME	DISTANCE	INTENSITY

REST DAY

MY DAY

FOOD JOURNAL

Breakfast

PROTEIN	FATS	CARBS	CALORIES

Lunch

PROTEIN	FATS	CARBS	CALORIES

Dinner

PROTEIN	FATS	CARBS	CALORIES

Snacks

PROTEIN	FATS	CARBS	CALORIES

WATER 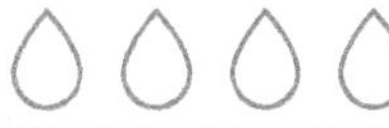

SLEEP (HRS) 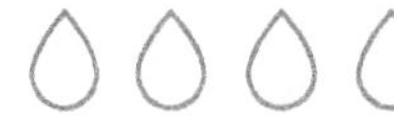

DAILY STEPS 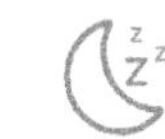

FOCUS

☐ Legs   ☐ Arms   ☐ Abs   ☐ Full body

STRENGTH

EXERCISE	SETS	REPS	WEIGHT

CARDIO

	TIME	DISTANCE	INTENSITY

REST DAY

MY DAY

DATE: _______________   M T W T F S S

FOOD JOURNAL

Breakfast

PROTEIN	FATS	CARBS	CALORIES

Lunch

PROTEIN	FATS	CARBS	CALORIES

Dinner

PROTEIN	FATS	CARBS	CALORIES

Snacks

PROTEIN	FATS	CARBS	CALORIES

WATER

○ ○ ○ ○ ○ ○ ○ ○

SLEEP (HRS)

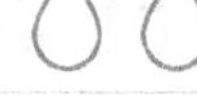

DAILY STEPS

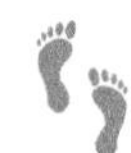

FOCUS

☐ Legs ☐ Arms ☐ Abs ☐ Full body

STRENGTH

EXERCISE	SETS	REPS	WEIGHT

CARDIO

	TIME	DISTANCE	INTENSITY

REST DAY

MY DAY

FOOD JOURNAL

DATE: / /

M T W T F S S

Breakfast

PROTEIN	FATS	CARBS	CALORIES

Lunch

PROTEIN	FATS	CARBS	CALORIES

Dinner

PROTEIN	FATS	CARBS	CALORIES

Snacks

PROTEIN	FATS	CARBS	CALORIES

WATER

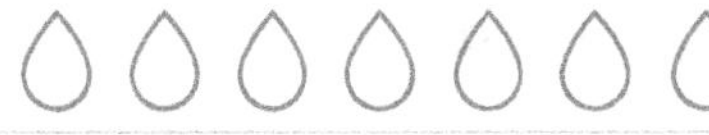

SLEEP (HRS)

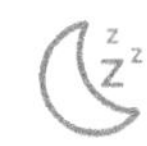

DAILY STEPS

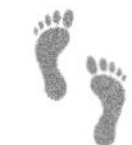

FOCUS

☐ Legs ☐ Arms ☐ Abs ☐ Full body

STRENGTH

EXERCISE	SETS	REPS	WEIGHT

CARDIO

	TIME	DISTANCE	INTENSITY

REST DAY

MY DAY

DATE: ______________________ M T W T F S S

FOOD JOURNAL

Breakfast

PROTEIN	FATS	CARBS	CALORIES

Lunch

PROTEIN	FATS	CARBS	CALORIES

Dinner

PROTEIN	FATS	CARBS	CALORIES

Snacks

PROTEIN	FATS	CARBS	CALORIES

WATER ○ ○ ○ ○ ○ ○ ○ ○

SLEEP (HRS)

DAILY STEPS

FOCUS

☐ Legs ☐ Arms ☐ Abs ☐ Full body

STRENGTH

EXERCISE	SETS	REPS	WEIGHT

CARDIO

	TIME	DISTANCE	INTENSITY

REST DAY

MY DAY

DATE: _______ / _______ / _______   M T W T F S S

FOOD JOURNAL

Breakfast

PROTEIN	FATS	CARBS	CALORIES

Lunch

PROTEIN	FATS	CARBS	CALORIES

Dinner

PROTEIN	FATS	CARBS	CALORIES

Snacks

PROTEIN	FATS	CARBS	CALORIES

WATER

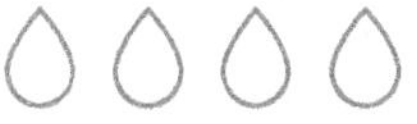 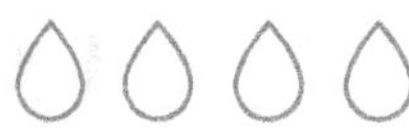

SLEEP (HRS)

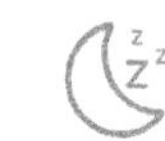

DAILY STEPS

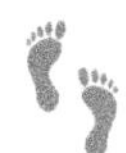

FOCUS

☐ Legs   ☐ Arms   ☐ Abs   ☐ Full body

STRENGTH

EXERCISE	SETS	REPS	WEIGHT

CARDIO

	TIME	DISTANCE	INTENSITY

REST DAY

MY DAY

FOOD JOURNAL

Breakfast

PROTEIN   FATS   CARBS   CALORIES

Lunch

PROTEIN   FATS   CARBS   CALORIES

Dinner

PROTEIN   FATS   CARBS   CALORIES

Snacks

PROTEIN   FATS   CARBS   CALORIES

WATER

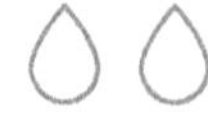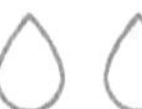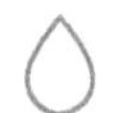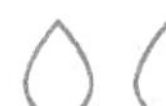

SLEEP (HRS)

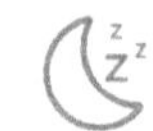

DAILY STEPS

FOCUS

☐ Legs   ☐ Arms   ☐ Abs   ☐ Full body

STRENGTH

EXERCISE	SETS	REPS	WEIGHT

CARDIO

	TIME	DISTANCE	INTENSITY

REST DAY

MY DAY

DATE: / /   M T W T F S S

FOOD JOURNAL

Breakfast

PROTEIN	FATS	CARBS	CALORIES

Lunch

PROTEIN	FATS	CARBS	CALORIES

Dinner

PROTEIN	FATS	CARBS	CALORIES

Snacks

PROTEIN	FATS	CARBS	CALORIES

WATER

SLEEP (HRS)

DAILY STEPS

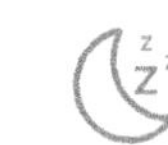

FOCUS

☐ Legs   ☐ Arms   ☐ Abs   ☐ Full body

STRENGTH

EXERCISE	SETS	REPS	WEIGHT

CARDIO

	TIME	DISTANCE	INTENSITY

REST DAY

MY DAY

DATE: / /   M T W T F S S

FOOD JOURNAL

Breakfast

PROTEIN	FATS	CARBS	CALORIES

Lunch

PROTEIN	FATS	CARBS	CALORIES

Dinner

PROTEIN	FATS	CARBS	CALORIES

Snacks

PROTEIN	FATS	CARBS	CALORIES

WATER

SLEEP (HRS)

DAILY STEPS

FOCUS

☐ Legs   ☐ Arms   ☐ Abs   ☐ Full body

STRENGTH

EXERCISE	SETS	REPS	WEIGHT

CARDIO

	TIME	DISTANCE	INTENSITY

REST DAY

MY DAY

DATE: / /   M T W T F S S

FOOD JOURNAL

Breakfast

PROTEIN	FATS	CARBS	CALORIES

Lunch

PROTEIN	FATS	CARBS	CALORIES

Dinner

PROTEIN	FATS	CARBS	CALORIES

Snacks

PROTEIN	FATS	CARBS	CALORIES

WATER

SLEEP (HRS)

DAILY STEPS

FOCUS

☐ Legs ☐ Arms ☐ Abs ☐ Full body

STRENGTH

EXERCISE	SETS	REPS	WEIGHT

CARDIO

	TIME	DISTANCE	INTENSITY

REST DAY

MY DAY

DATE: / /   M T W T F S S

FOOD JOURNAL

Breakfast

PROTEIN	FATS	CARBS	CALORIES

Lunch

PROTEIN	FATS	CARBS	CALORIES

Dinner

PROTEIN	FATS	CARBS	CALORIES

Snacks

PROTEIN	FATS	CARBS	CALORIES

WATER ○ ○ ○ ○ ○ ○ ○ ○

SLEEP (HRS)

DAILY STEPS

FOCUS

☐ Legs   ☐ Arms   ☐ Abs   ☐ Full body

STRENGTH

EXERCISE	SETS	REPS	WEIGHT

CARDIO

	TIME	DISTANCE	INTENSITY

REST DAY

MY DAY

FOOD JOURNAL

Breakfast

PROTEIN	FATS	CARBS	CALORIES

Lunch

PROTEIN	FATS	CARBS	CALORIES

Dinner

PROTEIN	FATS	CARBS	CALORIES

Snacks

PROTEIN	FATS	CARBS	CALORIES

DATE: / /

M T W T F S S

WATER

SLEEP (HRS)

DAILY STEPS

FOCUS

☐ Legs ☐ Arms ☐ Abs ☐ Full body

STRENGTH

EXERCISE	SETS	REPS	WEIGHT

CARDIO

	TIME	DISTANCE	INTENSITY

REST DAY

MY DAY

DATE: ___/___/___   M T W T F S S

FOOD JOURNAL

Breakfast

PROTEIN	FATS	CARBS	CALORIES

Lunch

PROTEIN	FATS	CARBS	CALORIES

Dinner

PROTEIN	FATS	CARBS	CALORIES

Snacks

PROTEIN	FATS	CARBS	CALORIES

WATER

○ ○ ○ ○ ○ ○ ○ ○

SLEEP (HRS)

DAILY STEPS

FOCUS

☐ Legs   ☐ Arms   ☐ Abs   ☐ Full body

STRENGTH

EXERCISE	SETS	REPS	WEIGHT

CARDIO

	TIME	DISTANCE	INTENSITY

REST DAY

MY DAY

FOOD JOURNAL

DATE: / /

M T W T F S S

Breakfast

PROTEIN	FATS	CARBS	CALORIES

Lunch

PROTEIN	FATS	CARBS	CALORIES

Dinner

PROTEIN	FATS	CARBS	CALORIES

Snacks

PROTEIN	FATS	CARBS	CALORIES

WATER

SLEEP (HRS)

DAILY STEPS

FOCUS

☐ Legs ☐ Arms ☐ Abs ☐ Full body

STRENGTH

EXERCISE	SETS	REPS	WEIGHT

CARDIO

	TIME	DISTANCE	INTENSITY

REST DAY

MY DAY

DATE: ____ / ____ / ____   M T W T F S S

FOOD JOURNAL

Breakfast

PROTEIN	FATS	CARBS	CALORIES

Lunch

PROTEIN	FATS	CARBS	CALORIES

Dinner

PROTEIN	FATS	CARBS	CALORIES

Snacks

PROTEIN	FATS	CARBS	CALORIES

WATER

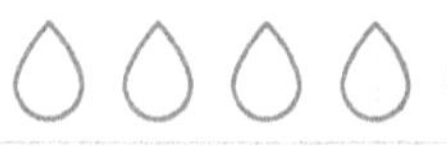

SLEEP (HRS)

DAILY STEPS

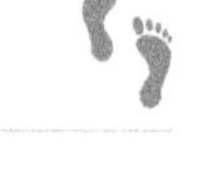

FOCUS

☐ Legs   ☐ Arms   ☐ Abs   ☐ Full body

STRENGTH

EXERCISE	SETS	REPS	WEIGHT

CARDIO

	TIME	DISTANCE	INTENSITY

REST DAY

MY DAY

DATE: / /   M T W T F S S

FOOD JOURNAL

Breakfast

PROTEIN	FATS	CARBS	CALORIES

Lunch

PROTEIN	FATS	CARBS	CALORIES

Dinner

PROTEIN	FATS	CARBS	CALORIES

Snacks

PROTEIN	FATS	CARBS	CALORIES

WATER

SLEEP (HRS)

DAILY STEPS

FOCUS

☐ Legs ☐ Arms ☐ Abs ☐ Full body

STRENGTH

EXERCISE	SETS	REPS	WEIGHT

CARDIO

	TIME	DISTANCE	INTENSITY

REST DAY

MY DAY

DATE: / /   M T W T F S S

FOOD JOURNAL

Breakfast

PROTEIN	FATS	CARBS	CALORIES

Lunch

PROTEIN	FATS	CARBS	CALORIES

Dinner

PROTEIN	FATS	CARBS	CALORIES

Snacks

PROTEIN	FATS	CARBS	CALORIES

WATER

SLEEP (HRS)

DAILY STEPS

FOCUS

☐ Legs ☐ Arms ☐ Abs ☐ Full body

STRENGTH

EXERCISE	SETS	REPS	WEIGHT

CARDIO

	TIME	DISTANCE	INTENSITY

REST DAY

MY DAY

DATE: _____ / _____ / _____   M T W T F S S

FOOD JOURNAL

Breakfast

PROTEIN	FATS	CARBS	CALORIES

Lunch

PROTEIN	FATS	CARBS	CALORIES

Dinner

PROTEIN	FATS	CARBS	CALORIES

Snacks

PROTEIN	FATS	CARBS	CALORIES

WATER

○ ○ ○ ○ ○ ○ ○ ○

SLEEP (HRS)

DAILY STEPS

FOCUS

☐ Legs   ☐ Arms   ☐ Abs   ☐ Full body

STRENGTH

EXERCISE	SETS	REPS	WEIGHT

CARDIO

	TIME	DISTANCE	INTENSITY

REST DAY

MY DAY

DATE: / /   M T W T F S S

FOOD JOURNAL

Breakfast

PROTEIN	FATS	CARBS	CALORIES

Lunch

PROTEIN	FATS	CARBS	CALORIES

Dinner

PROTEIN	FATS	CARBS	CALORIES

Snacks

PROTEIN	FATS	CARBS	CALORIES

WATER ◯ ◯ ◯ ◯ ◯ ◯ ◯ ◯

SLEEP (HRS)

DAILY STEPS

FOCUS

☐ Legs   ☐ Arms   ☐ Abs   ☐ Full body

STRENGTH

EXERCISE	SETS	REPS	WEIGHT

CARDIO

	TIME	DISTANCE	INTENSITY

REST DAY

MY DAY

DATE: / /   M T W T F S S

FOOD JOURNAL

Breakfast

PROTEIN	FATS	CARBS	CALORIES

Lunch

PROTEIN	FATS	CARBS	CALORIES

Dinner

PROTEIN	FATS	CARBS	CALORIES

Snacks

PROTEIN	FATS	CARBS	CALORIES

WATER

○ ○ ○ ○ ○ ○ ○ ○

SLEEP (HRS)

DAILY STEPS

FOCUS

☐ Legs ☐ Arms ☐ Abs ☐ Full body

STRENGTH

EXERCISE	SETS	REPS	WEIGHT

CARDIO

	TIME	DISTANCE	INTENSITY

REST DAY

MY DAY

DATE: _____ / _____ / _____   M T W T F S S

FOOD JOURNAL

Breakfast

PROTEIN	FATS	CARBS	CALORIES

Lunch

PROTEIN	FATS	CARBS	CALORIES

Dinner

PROTEIN	FATS	CARBS	CALORIES

Snacks

PROTEIN	FATS	CARBS	CALORIES

WATER ◇ ◇ ◇ ◇ ◇ ◇ ◇ ◇

SLEEP (HRS)

DAILY STEPS

FOCUS

☐ Legs   ☐ Arms   ☐ Abs   ☐ Full body

STRENGTH

EXERCISE	SETS	REPS	WEIGHT

CARDIO

	TIME	DISTANCE	INTENSITY

REST DAY

MY DAY

DATE: _______________   M T W T F S S

FOOD JOURNAL

Breakfast

PROTEIN	FATS	CARBS	CALORIES

Lunch

PROTEIN	FATS	CARBS	CALORIES

Dinner

PROTEIN	FATS	CARBS	CALORIES

Snacks

PROTEIN	FATS	CARBS	CALORIES

WATER

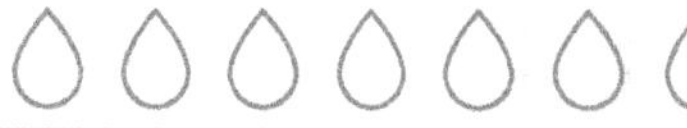

SLEEP (HRS)

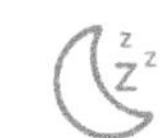

DAILY STEPS

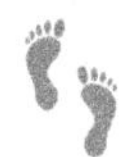

FOCUS

☐ Legs   ☐ Arms   ☐ Abs   ☐ Full body

STRENGTH

EXERCISE	SETS	REPS	WEIGHT

CARDIO

	TIME	DISTANCE	INTENSITY

REST DAY

MY DAY

DATE: ___________   M T W T F S S

FOOD JOURNAL

Breakfast

PROTEIN	FATS	CARBS	CALORIES

Lunch

PROTEIN	FATS	CARBS	CALORIES

Dinner

PROTEIN	FATS	CARBS	CALORIES

Snacks

PROTEIN	FATS	CARBS	CALORIES

WATER

SLEEP (HRS)

DAILY STEPS

FOCUS

☐ Legs   ☐ Arms   ☐ Abs   ☐ Full body

STRENGTH

EXERCISE	SETS	REPS	WEIGHT

CARDIO

	TIME	DISTANCE	INTENSITY

REST DAY

MY DAY

FOOD JOURNAL

DATE: / /   M T W T F S S

Breakfast

PROTEIN	FATS	CARBS	CALORIES

Lunch

PROTEIN	FATS	CARBS	CALORIES

Dinner

PROTEIN	FATS	CARBS	CALORIES

Snacks

PROTEIN	FATS	CARBS	CALORIES

WATER ◇ ◇ ◇ ◇ ◇ ◇ ◇ ◇

SLEEP (HRS)

DAILY STEPS

FOCUS

☐ Legs   ☐ Arms   ☐ Abs   ☐ Full body

STRENGTH

EXERCISE	SETS	REPS	WEIGHT

CARDIO

	TIME	DISTANCE	INTENSITY

REST DAY

MY DAY

DATE: / /

M T W T F S S

FOOD JOURNAL

Breakfast

PROTEIN	FATS	CARBS	CALORIES

Lunch

PROTEIN	FATS	CARBS	CALORIES

Dinner

PROTEIN	FATS	CARBS	CALORIES

Snacks

PROTEIN	FATS	CARBS	CALORIES

WATER

SLEEP (HRS)

DAILY STEPS

FOCUS

☐ Legs ☐ Arms ☐ Abs ☐ Full body

STRENGTH

EXERCISE	SETS	REPS	WEIGHT

CARDIO

	TIME	DISTANCE	INTENSITY

REST DAY

MY DAY

DATE: / /   M T W T F S S

FOOD JOURNAL

Breakfast

PROTEIN	FATS	CARBS	CALORIES

Lunch

PROTEIN	FATS	CARBS	CALORIES

Dinner

PROTEIN	FATS	CARBS	CALORIES

Snacks

PROTEIN	FATS	CARBS	CALORIES

WATER ◊ ◊ ◊ ◊ ◊ ◊ ◊ ◊

SLEEP (HRS)

DAILY STEPS

FOCUS

☐ Legs ☐ Arms ☐ Abs ☐ Full body

STRENGTH

EXERCISE	SETS	REPS	WEIGHT

CARDIO

	TIME	DISTANCE	INTENSITY

REST DAY

MY DAY

DATE: _____ / _____ / _____   M T W T F S S

FOOD JOURNAL

Breakfast

PROTEIN	FATS	CARBS	CALORIES

Lunch

PROTEIN	FATS	CARBS	CALORIES

Dinner

PROTEIN	FATS	CARBS	CALORIES

Snacks

PROTEIN	FATS	CARBS	CALORIES

WATER

◊ ◊ ◊ ◊ ◊ ◊ ◊ ◊

SLEEP (HRS)

DAILY STEPS

FOCUS

☐ Legs   ☐ Arms   ☐ Abs   ☐ Full body

STRENGTH

EXERCISE	SETS	REPS	WEIGHT

CARDIO

	TIME	DISTANCE	INTENSITY

REST DAY

MY DAY

FOOD JOURNAL

Breakfast

PROTEIN	FATS	CARBS	CALORIES

Lunch

PROTEIN	FATS	CARBS	CALORIES

Dinner

PROTEIN	FATS	CARBS	CALORIES

Snacks

PROTEIN	FATS	CARBS	CALORIES

DATE:

M T W T F S S

WATER

SLEEP (HRS)

DAILY STEPS

FOCUS

☐ Legs   ☐ Arms   ☐ Abs   ☐ Full body

STRENGTH

EXERCISE	SETS	REPS	WEIGHT

CARDIO

	TIME	DISTANCE	INTENSITY

REST DAY

MY DAY

DATE: / /

M T W T F S S

FOOD JOURNAL

Breakfast

PROTEIN	FATS	CARBS	CALORIES

Lunch

PROTEIN	FATS	CARBS	CALORIES

Dinner

PROTEIN	FATS	CARBS	CALORIES

Snacks

PROTEIN	FATS	CARBS	CALORIES

WATER

SLEEP (HRS)

DAILY STEPS

FOCUS

☐ Legs ☐ Arms ☐ Abs ☐ Full body

STRENGTH

EXERCISE	SETS	REPS	WEIGHT

CARDIO

	TIME	DISTANCE	INTENSITY

REST DAY

MY DAY

DATE: ___/___/___   M T W T F S S

FOOD JOURNAL

Breakfast

PROTEIN	FATS	CARBS	CALORIES

Lunch

PROTEIN	FATS	CARBS	CALORIES

Dinner

PROTEIN	FATS	CARBS	CALORIES

Snacks

PROTEIN	FATS	CARBS	CALORIES

WATER ◇ ◇ ◇ ◇ ◇ ◇ ◇ ◇

SLEEP (HRS)

DAILY STEPS

FOCUS

☐ Legs   ☐ Arms   ☐ Abs   ☐ Full body

STRENGTH

EXERCISE	SETS	REPS	WEIGHT

CARDIO

	TIME	DISTANCE	INTENSITY

REST DAY

MY DAY

FOOD JOURNAL

Breakfast

PROTEIN	FATS	CARBS	CALORIES

Lunch

PROTEIN	FATS	CARBS	CALORIES

Dinner

PROTEIN	FATS	CARBS	CALORIES

Snacks

PROTEIN	FATS	CARBS	CALORIES

WATER

SLEEP (HRS)

DAILY STEPS

FOCUS

☐ Legs ☐ Arms ☐ Abs ☐ Full body

STRENGTH

EXERCISE	SETS	REPS	WEIGHT

CARDIO

	TIME	DISTANCE	INTENSITY

REST DAY

MY DAY

DATE: _____ / _____ / _____   M T W T F S S

FOOD JOURNAL

Breakfast

PROTEIN	FATS	CARBS	CALORIES

Lunch

PROTEIN	FATS	CARBS	CALORIES

Dinner

PROTEIN	FATS	CARBS	CALORIES

Snacks

PROTEIN	FATS	CARBS	CALORIES

WATER ◌ ◌ ◌ ◌ ◌ ◌ ◌ ◌

SLEEP (HRS)

DAILY STEPS

FOCUS

☐ Legs   ☐ Arms   ☐ Abs   ☐ Full body

STRENGTH

EXERCISE	SETS	REPS	WEIGHT

CARDIO

	TIME	DISTANCE	INTENSITY

REST DAY

MY DAY

DATE: / /　　　　　　M T W T F S S

FOOD JOURNAL

Breakfast

PROTEIN	FATS	CARBS	CALORIES

Lunch

PROTEIN	FATS	CARBS	CALORIES

Dinner

PROTEIN	FATS	CARBS	CALORIES

Snacks

PROTEIN	FATS	CARBS	CALORIES

WATER

SLEEP (HRS)

DAILY STEPS

FOCUS

☐ Legs ☐ Arms ☐ Abs ☐ Full body

STRENGTH

EXERCISE	SETS	REPS	WEIGHT

CARDIO

	TIME	DISTANCE	INTENSITY

REST DAY

MY DAY

DATE: / / M T W T F S S

FOOD JOURNAL

Breakfast

PROTEIN	FATS	CARBS	CALORIES

Lunch

PROTEIN	FATS	CARBS	CALORIES

Dinner

PROTEIN	FATS	CARBS	CALORIES

Snacks

PROTEIN	FATS	CARBS	CALORIES

WATER ◯ ◯ ◯ ◯ ◯ ◯ ◯ ◯

SLEEP (HRS)

DAILY STEPS

FOCUS

☐ Legs ☐ Arms ☐ Abs ☐ Full body

STRENGTH

EXERCISE	SETS	REPS	WEIGHT

CARDIO

	TIME	DISTANCE	INTENSITY

REST DAY

MY DAY

DATE: ___/___/___   M T W T F S S

FOOD JOURNAL

Breakfast

PROTEIN	FATS	CARBS	CALORIES

Lunch

PROTEIN	FATS	CARBS	CALORIES

Dinner

PROTEIN	FATS	CARBS	CALORIES

Snacks

PROTEIN	FATS	CARBS	CALORIES

WATER

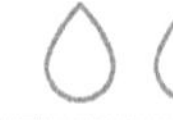   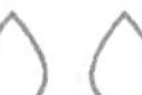

SLEEP (HRS)

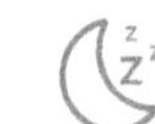

DAILY STEPS

FOCUS

☐ Legs   ☐ Arms   ☐ Abs   ☐ Full body

STRENGTH

EXERCISE		SETS	REPS	WEIGHT

CARDIO

	TIME	DISTANCE	INTENSITY

REST DAY

MY DAY

DATE: _____ / _____ / _____   M T W T F S S

FOOD JOURNAL

Breakfast

PROTEIN	FATS	CARBS	CALORIES

Lunch

PROTEIN	FATS	CARBS	CALORIES

Dinner

PROTEIN	FATS	CARBS	CALORIES

Snacks

PROTEIN	FATS	CARBS	CALORIES

WATER ◇ ◇ ◇ ◇ ◇ ◇ ◇ ◇

SLEEP (HRS)

DAILY STEPS

FOCUS

☐ Legs ☐ Arms ☐ Abs ☐ Full body

STRENGTH

EXERCISE	SETS	REPS	WEIGHT

CARDIO

	TIME	DISTANCE	INTENSITY

REST DAY

MY DAY

DATE: / /   M T W T F S S

FOOD JOURNAL

Breakfast

PROTEIN	FATS	CARBS	CALORIES

Lunch

PROTEIN	FATS	CARBS	CALORIES

Dinner

PROTEIN	FATS	CARBS	CALORIES

Snacks

PROTEIN	FATS	CARBS	CALORIES

WATER

○ ○ ○ ○ ○ ○ ○ ○

SLEEP (HRS)

DAILY STEPS

FOCUS

☐ Legs   ☐ Arms   ☐ Abs   ☐ Full body

STRENGTH

EXERCISE	SETS	REPS	WEIGHT

CARDIO

	TIME	DISTANCE	INTENSITY

REST DAY

MY DAY

FOOD JOURNAL

Breakfast

PROTEIN	FATS	CARBS	CALORIES

Lunch

PROTEIN	FATS	CARBS	CALORIES

Dinner

PROTEIN	FATS	CARBS	CALORIES

Snacks

PROTEIN	FATS	CARBS	CALORIES

DATE: M T W T F S S

WATER

SLEEP (HRS)

DAILY STEPS

FOCUS

☐ Legs ☐ Arms ☐ Abs ☐ Full body

STRENGTH

EXERCISE	SETS	REPS	WEIGHT

CARDIO

	TIME	DISTANCE	INTENSITY

REST DAY

MY DAY

DATE: _______________   M T W T F S S

FOOD JOURNAL

Breakfast

PROTEIN	FATS	CARBS	CALORIES

Lunch

PROTEIN	FATS	CARBS	CALORIES

Dinner

PROTEIN	FATS	CARBS	CALORIES

Snacks

PROTEIN	FATS	CARBS	CALORIES

WATER

SLEEP (HRS)

DAILY STEPS

FOCUS

☐ Legs   ☐ Arms   ☐ Abs   ☐ Full body

STRENGTH

EXERCISE	SETS	REPS	WEIGHT

CARDIO

	TIME	DISTANCE	INTENSITY

REST DAY

MY DAY

DATE: ___/___/___   M T W T F S S

FOOD JOURNAL

Breakfast

PROTEIN	FATS	CARBS	CALORIES

Lunch

PROTEIN	FATS	CARBS	CALORIES

Dinner

PROTEIN	FATS	CARBS	CALORIES

Snacks

PROTEIN	FATS	CARBS	CALORIES

WATER

SLEEP (HRS)

DAILY STEPS

FOCUS

☐ Legs ☐ Arms ☐ Abs ☐ Full body

STRENGTH

EXERCISE	SETS	REPS	WEIGHT

CARDIO

	TIME	DISTANCE	INTENSITY

REST DAY

MY DAY

DATE: _______________ M T W T F S S

FOOD JOURNAL

Breakfast

PROTEIN	FATS	CARBS	CALORIES

Lunch

PROTEIN	FATS	CARBS	CALORIES

Dinner

PROTEIN	FATS	CARBS	CALORIES

Snacks

PROTEIN	FATS	CARBS	CALORIES

WATER

SLEEP (HRS)

DAILY STEPS

FOCUS

☐ Legs ☐ Arms ☐ Abs ☐ Full body

STRENGTH

EXERCISE	SETS	REPS	WEIGHT

CARDIO

	TIME	DISTANCE	INTENSITY

REST DAY

MY DAY

DATE: / /　　　　　　　M T W T F S S

FOOD JOURNAL

Breakfast

PROTEIN	FATS	CARBS	CALORIES

Lunch

PROTEIN	FATS	CARBS	CALORIES

Dinner

PROTEIN	FATS	CARBS	CALORIES

Snacks

PROTEIN	FATS	CARBS	CALORIES

WATER

SLEEP (HRS)

DAILY STEPS

FOCUS

☐ Legs　　☐ Arms　　☐ Abs　　☐ Full body

STRENGTH

EXERCISE	SETS	REPS	WEIGHT

CARDIO

	TIME	DISTANCE	INTENSITY

REST DAY

MY DAY

DATE: / /   M T W T F S S

FOOD JOURNAL

Breakfast

PROTEIN	FATS	CARBS	CALORIES

Lunch

PROTEIN	FATS	CARBS	CALORIES

Dinner

PROTEIN	FATS	CARBS	CALORIES

Snacks

PROTEIN	FATS	CARBS	CALORIES

WATER

SLEEP (HRS)

DAILY STEPS

FOCUS

☐ Legs ☐ Arms ☐ Abs ☐ Full body

STRENGTH

EXERCISE	SETS	REPS	WEIGHT

CARDIO

	TIME	DISTANCE	INTENSITY

REST DAY

MY DAY

DATE: _______________   M T W T F S S

FOOD JOURNAL

Breakfast

PROTEIN	FATS	CARBS	CALORIES

Lunch

PROTEIN	FATS	CARBS	CALORIES

Dinner

PROTEIN	FATS	CARBS	CALORIES

Snacks

PROTEIN	FATS	CARBS	CALORIES

WATER ○ ○ ○ ○ ○ ○ ○ ○

SLEEP (HRS)

DAILY STEPS

FOCUS

☐ Legs   ☐ Arms   ☐ Abs   ☐ Full body

STRENGTH

EXERCISE	SETS	REPS	WEIGHT

CARDIO

	TIME	DISTANCE	INTENSITY

REST DAY

MY DAY

DATE: / /   M T W T F S S

FOOD JOURNAL

Breakfast

PROTEIN	FATS	CARBS	CALORIES

Lunch

PROTEIN	FATS	CARBS	CALORIES

Dinner

PROTEIN	FATS	CARBS	CALORIES

Snacks

PROTEIN	FATS	CARBS	CALORIES

WATER ○○○○○○○○

SLEEP (HRS)

DAILY STEPS

FOCUS

☐ Legs ☐ Arms ☐ Abs ☐ Full body

STRENGTH

EXERCISE	SETS	REPS	WEIGHT

CARDIO

	TIME	DISTANCE	INTENSITY

REST DAY

MY DAY

DATE: _____ / _____ / _____   M T W T F S S

FOOD JOURNAL

Breakfast

PROTEIN	FATS	CARBS	CALORIES

Lunch

PROTEIN	FATS	CARBS	CALORIES

Dinner

PROTEIN	FATS	CARBS	CALORIES

Snacks

PROTEIN	FATS	CARBS	CALORIES

WATER

◇ ◇ ◇ ◇ ◇ ◇ ◇ ◇

SLEEP (HRS)

DAILY STEPS

FOCUS

☐ Legs   ☐ Arms   ☐ Abs   ☐ Full body

STRENGTH

EXERCISE	SETS	REPS	WEIGHT

CARDIO

	TIME	DISTANCE	INTENSITY

REST DAY

MY DAY

DATE: _______________   M T W T F S S

FOOD JOURNAL

Breakfast

PROTEIN	FATS	CARBS	CALORIES

Lunch

PROTEIN	FATS	CARBS	CALORIES

Dinner

PROTEIN	FATS	CARBS	CALORIES

Snacks

PROTEIN	FATS	CARBS	CALORIES

WATER ○ ○ ○ ○ ○ ○ ○ ○

SLEEP (HRS)

DAILY STEPS

FOCUS

☐ Legs   ☐ Arms   ☐ Abs   ☐ Full body

STRENGTH

EXERCISE	SETS	REPS	WEIGHT

CARDIO

	TIME	DISTANCE	INTENSITY

REST DAY

MY DAY

DATE: / /   M T W T F S S

FOOD JOURNAL

Breakfast

PROTEIN	FATS	CARBS	CALORIES

Lunch

PROTEIN	FATS	CARBS	CALORIES

Dinner

PROTEIN	FATS	CARBS	CALORIES

Snacks

PROTEIN	FATS	CARBS	CALORIES

WATER

⬡ ⬡ ⬡ ⬡ ⬡ ⬡ ⬡ ⬡

SLEEP (HRS)

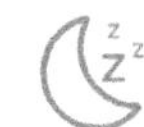

DAILY STEPS

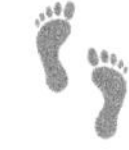

FOCUS

☐ Legs   ☐ Arms   ☐ Abs   ☐ Full body

STRENGTH

EXERCISE	SETS	REPS	WEIGHT

CARDIO

	TIME	DISTANCE	INTENSITY

REST DAY

MY DAY

DATE: / / M T W T F S S

FOOD JOURNAL

Breakfast

PROTEIN	FATS	CARBS	CALORIES

Lunch

PROTEIN	FATS	CARBS	CALORIES

Dinner

PROTEIN	FATS	CARBS	CALORIES

Snacks

PROTEIN	FATS	CARBS	CALORIES

WATER

SLEEP (HRS)

DAILY STEPS

FOCUS

☐ Legs ☐ Arms ☐ Abs ☐ Full body

STRENGTH

EXERCISE	SETS	REPS	WEIGHT

CARDIO

	TIME	DISTANCE	INTENSITY

REST DAY

MY DAY

FOOD JOURNAL

DATE: ___________   M T W T F S S

Breakfast

PROTEIN	FATS	CARBS	CALORIES

Lunch

PROTEIN	FATS	CARBS	CALORIES

Dinner

PROTEIN	FATS	CARBS	CALORIES

Snacks

PROTEIN	FATS	CARBS	CALORIES

WATER ○ ○ ○ ○ ○ ○ ○ ○

SLEEP (HRS)

DAILY STEPS

FOCUS

☐ Legs   ☐ Arms   ☐ Abs   ☐ Full body

STRENGTH

EXERCISE	SETS	REPS	WEIGHT

CARDIO

	TIME	DISTANCE	INTENSITY

REST DAY

MY DAY

FOOD JOURNAL

Breakfast

PROTEIN   FATS   CARBS   CALORIES

Lunch

PROTEIN   FATS   CARBS   CALORIES

Dinner

PROTEIN   FATS   CARBS   CALORIES

Snacks

PROTEIN   FATS   CARBS   CALORIES

DATE: / /

M T W T F S S

WATER

○ ○ ○ ○ ○ ○ ○ ○

SLEEP (HRS)

DAILY STEPS

FOCUS

☐ Legs   ☐ Arms   ☐ Abs   ☐ Full body

STRENGTH

EXERCISE	SETS	REPS	WEIGHT

CARDIO

	TIME	DISTANCE	INTENSITY

REST DAY

MY DAY

DATE: _________ / _________   M T W T F S S

FOOD JOURNAL

Breakfast

PROTEIN	FATS	CARBS	CALORIES

Lunch

PROTEIN	FATS	CARBS	CALORIES

Dinner

PROTEIN	FATS	CARBS	CALORIES

Snacks

PROTEIN	FATS	CARBS	CALORIES

WATER ○ ○ ○ ○ ○ ○ ○ ○

SLEEP (HRS)

DAILY STEPS

FOCUS

☐ Legs   ☐ Arms   ☐ Abs   ☐ Full body

STRENGTH

EXERCISE	SETS	REPS	WEIGHT

CARDIO

	TIME	DISTANCE	INTENSITY

REST DAY

MY DAY

DATE: / /   M T W T F S S

FOOD JOURNAL

Breakfast

PROTEIN	FATS	CARBS	CALORIES

Lunch

PROTEIN	FATS	CARBS	CALORIES

Dinner

PROTEIN	FATS	CARBS	CALORIES

Snacks

PROTEIN	FATS	CARBS	CALORIES

WATER

SLEEP (HRS)

DAILY STEPS

FOCUS

☐ Legs ☐ Arms ☐ Abs ☐ Full body

STRENGTH

EXERCISE	SETS	REPS	WEIGHT

CARDIO

	TIME	DISTANCE	INTENSITY

REST DAY

MY DAY

DATE: ___/___/___   M T W T F S S

FOOD JOURNAL

Breakfast

PROTEIN	FATS	CARBS	CALORIES

Lunch

PROTEIN	FATS	CARBS	CALORIES

Dinner

PROTEIN	FATS	CARBS	CALORIES

Snacks

PROTEIN	FATS	CARBS	CALORIES

WATER 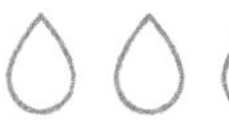 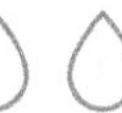 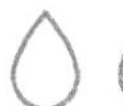 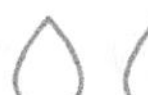

SLEEP (HRS) 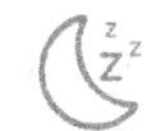

DAILY STEPS 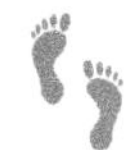

FOCUS

☐ Legs ☐ Arms ☐ Abs ☐ Full body

STRENGTH

EXERCISE	SETS	REPS	WEIGHT

CARDIO

	TIME	DISTANCE	INTENSITY

REST DAY

MY DAY

DATE:

FOOD JOURNAL

Breakfast

PROTEIN	FATS	CARBS	CALORIES

Lunch

PROTEIN	FATS	CARBS	CALORIES

Dinner

PROTEIN	FATS	CARBS	CALORIES

Snacks

PROTEIN	FATS	CARBS	CALORIES

WATER

SLEEP (HRS)

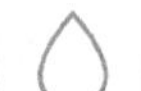

DAILY STEPS

FOCUS

☐ Legs   ☐ Arms   ☐ Abs   ☐ Full body

STRENGTH

EXERCISE	SETS	REPS	WEIGHT

CARDIO

	TIME	DISTANCE	INTENSITY

MY DAY

DATE: /   /   M T W T F S S

FOOD JOURNAL

Breakfast

PROTEIN	FATS	CARBS	CALORIES

Lunch

PROTEIN	FATS	CARBS	CALORIES

Dinner

PROTEIN	FATS	CARBS	CALORIES

Snacks

PROTEIN	FATS	CARBS	CALORIES

WATER ◯ ◯ ◯ ◯ ◯ ◯ ◯ ◯

SLEEP (HRS)

DAILY STEPS

FOCUS

☐ Legs ☐ Arms ☐ Abs ☐ Full body

STRENGTH

EXERCISE	SETS	REPS	WEIGHT

CARDIO

	TIME	DISTANCE	INTENSITY

REST DAY

MY DAY

DATE: / /

M T W T F S S

FOOD JOURNAL

Breakfast

PROTEIN	FATS	CARBS	CALORIES

Lunch

PROTEIN	FATS	CARBS	CALORIES

Dinner

PROTEIN	FATS	CARBS	CALORIES

Snacks

PROTEIN	FATS	CARBS	CALORIES

WATER

SLEEP (HRS)

DAILY STEPS

FOCUS

Legs	Arms	Abs	Full body

STRENGTH

EXERCISE	SETS	REPS	WEIGHT

CARDIO

	TIME	DISTANCE	INTENSITY

REST DAY

MY DAY

DATE: / /   M T W T F S S

FOOD JOURNAL

Breakfast

PROTEIN	FATS	CARBS	CALORIES

Lunch

PROTEIN	FATS	CARBS	CALORIES

Dinner

PROTEIN	FATS	CARBS	CALORIES

Snacks

PROTEIN	FATS	CARBS	CALORIES

WATER ○ ○ ○ ○ ○ ○ ○ ○

SLEEP (HRS)

DAILY STEPS

FOCUS

☐ Legs   ☐ Arms   ☐ Abs   ☐ Full body

STRENGTH

EXERCISE	SETS	REPS	WEIGHT

CARDIO

	TIME	DISTANCE	INTENSITY

REST DAY

MY DAY

DATE: / /

M T W T F S S

FOOD JOURNAL

Breakfast

PROTEIN	FATS	CARBS	CALORIES

Lunch

PROTEIN	FATS	CARBS	CALORIES

Dinner

PROTEIN	FATS	CARBS	CALORIES

Snacks

PROTEIN	FATS	CARBS	CALORIES

WATER

◇ ◇ ◇ ◇ ◇ ◇ ◇ ◇

SLEEP (HRS)

DAILY STEPS

FOCUS

☐ Legs ☐ Arms ☐ Abs ☐ Full body

STRENGTH

EXERCISE	SETS	REPS	WEIGHT

CARDIO

	TIME	DISTANCE	INTENSITY

REST DAY

MY DAY

DATE: ___________ M T W T F S S

FOOD JOURNAL

Breakfast

PROTEIN	FATS	CARBS	CALORIES

Lunch

PROTEIN	FATS	CARBS	CALORIES

Dinner

PROTEIN	FATS	CARBS	CALORIES

Snacks

PROTEIN	FATS	CARBS	CALORIES

WATER
◇ ◇ ◇ ◇ ◇ ◇ ◇ ◇

SLEEP (HRS)

DAILY STEPS

FOCUS

☐ Legs ☐ Arms ☐ Abs ☐ Full body

STRENGTH

EXERCISE	SETS	REPS	WEIGHT

CARDIO

	TIME	DISTANCE	INTENSITY

REST DAY

MY DAY

DATE: / / M T W T F S S

FOOD JOURNAL

Breakfast

PROTEIN	FATS	CARBS	CALORIES

Lunch

PROTEIN	FATS	CARBS	CALORIES

Dinner

PROTEIN	FATS	CARBS	CALORIES

Snacks

PROTEIN	FATS	CARBS	CALORIES

WATER

SLEEP (HRS)

DAILY STEPS

FOCUS

☐ Legs ☐ Arms ☐ Abs ☐ Full body

STRENGTH

EXERCISE	SETS	REPS	WEIGHT

CARDIO

	TIME	DISTANCE	INTENSITY

REST DAY

MY DAY

FOOD JOURNAL

DATE: _______________ M T W T F S S

Breakfast

PROTEIN	FATS	CARBS	CALORIES

Lunch

PROTEIN	FATS	CARBS	CALORIES

Dinner

PROTEIN	FATS	CARBS	CALORIES

Snacks

PROTEIN	FATS	CARBS	CALORIES

WATER

SLEEP (HRS)

DAILY STEPS

FOCUS

☐ Legs   ☐ Arms   ☐ Abs   ☐ Full body

STRENGTH

EXERCISE	SETS	REPS	WEIGHT

CARDIO

	TIME	DISTANCE	INTENSITY

REST DAY

MY DAY

DATE: ______________   M T W T F S S

FOOD JOURNAL

Breakfast

PROTEIN	FATS	CARBS	CALORIES

Lunch

PROTEIN	FATS	CARBS	CALORIES

Dinner

PROTEIN	FATS	CARBS	CALORIES

Snacks

PROTEIN	FATS	CARBS	CALORIES

WATER ○ ○ ○ ○ ○ ○ ○ ○

SLEEP (HRS)

DAILY STEPS

FOCUS

☐ Legs   ☐ Arms   ☐ Abs   ☐ Full body

STRENGTH

EXERCISE	SETS	REPS	WEIGHT

CARDIO

	TIME	DISTANCE	INTENSITY

REST DAY

MY DAY

DATE: / / M T W T F S S

FOOD JOURNAL

Breakfast

PROTEIN | FATS | CARBS | CALORIES

Lunch

PROTEIN | FATS | CARBS | CALORIES

Dinner

PROTEIN | FATS | CARBS | CALORIES

Snacks

PROTEIN | FATS | CARBS | CALORIES

WATER

SLEEP (HRS)

DAILY STEPS

FOCUS

☐ Legs ☐ Arms ☐ Abs ☐ Full body

STRENGTH

EXERCISE	SETS	REPS	WEIGHT

CARDIO

	TIME	DISTANCE	INTENSITY

REST DAY

MY DAY

DATE: _______ / _______

M T W T F S S

FOOD JOURNAL

Breakfast

PROTEIN	FATS	CARBS	CALORIES

Lunch

PROTEIN	FATS	CARBS	CALORIES

Dinner

PROTEIN	FATS	CARBS	CALORIES

Snacks

PROTEIN	FATS	CARBS	CALORIES

WATER

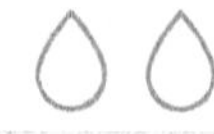 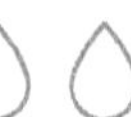 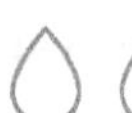 ○ ○ ○ ○ ○ ○ ○ ○

SLEEP (HRS)

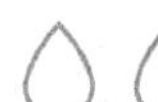

DAILY STEPS

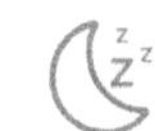

FOCUS

☐ Legs ☐ Arms ☐ Abs ☐ Full body

STRENGTH

EXERCISE	SETS	REPS	WEIGHT

CARDIO

	TIME	DISTANCE	INTENSITY

REST DAY

MY DAY

DATE: _____________   M T W T F S S

FOOD JOURNAL

Breakfast

PROTEIN	FATS	CARBS	CALORIES

Lunch

PROTEIN	FATS	CARBS	CALORIES

Dinner

PROTEIN	FATS	CARBS	CALORIES

Snacks

PROTEIN	FATS	CARBS	CALORIES

WATER ○○○○○○○○

SLEEP (HRS)

DAILY STEPS

FOCUS

☐ Legs   ☐ Arms   ☐ Abs   ☐ Full body

STRENGTH

EXERCISE	SETS	REPS	WEIGHT

CARDIO

	TIME	DISTANCE	INTENSITY

REST DAY

MY DAY

DATE: _____ / _____ / _____   M T W T F S S

FOOD JOURNAL

Breakfast

PROTEIN	FATS	CARBS	CALORIES

Lunch

PROTEIN	FATS	CARBS	CALORIES

Dinner

PROTEIN	FATS	CARBS	CALORIES

Snacks

PROTEIN	FATS	CARBS	CALORIES

WATER 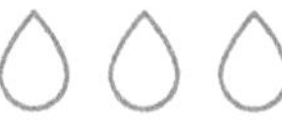 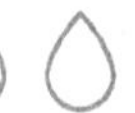 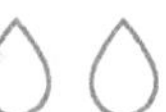 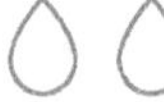

SLEEP (HRS) 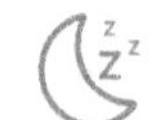

DAILY STEPS

FOCUS

☐ Legs   ☐ Arms   ☐ Abs   ☐ Full body

STRENGTH

EXERCISE	SETS	REPS	WEIGHT

CARDIO

	TIME	DISTANCE	INTENSITY

REST DAY

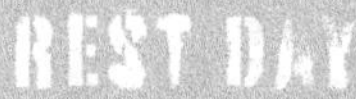

MY DAY

DATE: / / M T W T F S S

FOOD JOURNAL

Breakfast

PROTEIN	FATS	CARBS	CALORIES

Lunch

PROTEIN	FATS	CARBS	CALORIES

Dinner

PROTEIN	FATS	CARBS	CALORIES

Snacks

PROTEIN	FATS	CARBS	CALORIES

WATER

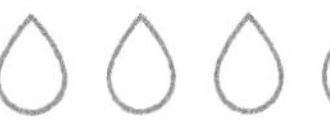 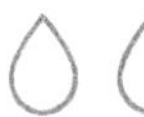 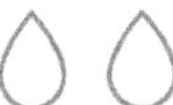

SLEEP (HRS)

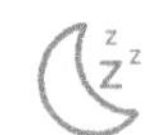

DAILY STEPS

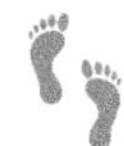

FOCUS

- [ ] Legs
- [ ] Arms
- [ ] Abs
- [ ] Full body

STRENGTH

EXERCISE	SETS	REPS	WEIGHT

CARDIO

	TIME	DISTANCE	INTENSITY

REST DAY

MY DAY

DATE: M T W T F S S

FOOD JOURNAL

Breakfast

PROTEIN	FATS	CARBS	CALORIES

Lunch

PROTEIN	FATS	CARBS	CALORIES

Dinner

PROTEIN	FATS	CARBS	CALORIES

Snacks

PROTEIN	FATS	CARBS	CALORIES

WATER

SLEEP (HRS)

DAILY STEPS

FOCUS

☐ Legs   ☐ Arms   ☐ Abs   ☐ Full body

STRENGTH

EXERCISE	SETS	REPS	WEIGHT

CARDIO

	TIME	DISTANCE	INTENSITY

REST DAY

MY DAY

DATE: _______________   M T W T F S S

FOOD JOURNAL

Breakfast

PROTEIN	FATS	CARBS	CALORIES

Lunch

PROTEIN	FATS	CARBS	CALORIES

Dinner

PROTEIN	FATS	CARBS	CALORIES

Snacks

PROTEIN	FATS	CARBS	CALORIES

WATER

○ ○ ○ ○ ○ ○ ○ ○

SLEEP (HRS)

DAILY STEPS

FOCUS

☐ Legs   ☐ Arms   ☐ Abs   ☐ Full body

STRENGTH

EXERCISE	SETS	REPS	WEIGHT

CARDIO

	TIME	DISTANCE	INTENSITY

REST DAY

MY DAY

M T W T F S S

FOOD JOURNAL

Breakfast

PROTEIN	FATS	CARBS	CALORIES

Lunch

PROTEIN	FATS	CARBS	CALORIES

Dinner

PROTEIN	FATS	CARBS	CALORIES

Snacks

PROTEIN	FATS	CARBS	CALORIES

WATER

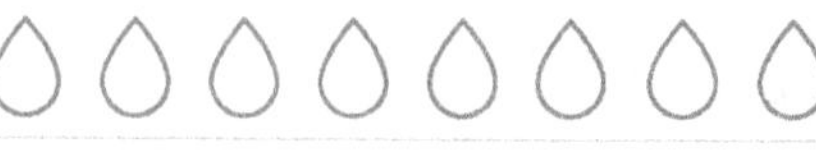

SLEEP (HRS)

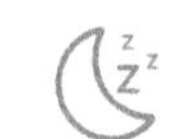

DAILY STEPS

FOCUS

☐ Legs ☐ Arms ☐ Abs ☐ Full body

STRENGTH

EXERCISE	SETS	REPS	WEIGHT

CARDIO

	TIME	DISTANCE	INTENSITY

REST DAY

MY DAY

DATE: M T W T F S S

FOOD JOURNAL

Breakfast

PROTEIN	FATS	CARBS	CALORIES

Lunch

PROTEIN	FATS	CARBS	CALORIES

Dinner

PROTEIN	FATS	CARBS	CALORIES

Snacks

PROTEIN	FATS	CARBS	CALORIES

WATER

SLEEP (HRS)

DAILY STEPS

FOCUS

- ☐ Legs
- ☐ Arms
- ☐ Abs
- ☐ Full body

STRENGTH

EXERCISE	SETS	REPS	WEIGHT

CARDIO

	TIME	DISTANCE	INTENSITY

REST DAY

MY DAY

DATE: ___________________   M T W T F S S

FOOD JOURNAL

Breakfast

PROTEIN	FATS	CARBS	CALORIES

Lunch

PROTEIN	FATS	CARBS	CALORIES

Dinner

PROTEIN	FATS	CARBS	CALORIES

Snacks

PROTEIN	FATS	CARBS	CALORIES

WATER

○ ○ ○ ○ ○ ○ ○ ○

SLEEP (HRS)

DAILY STEPS

FOCUS

☐ Legs ☐ Arms ☐ Abs ☐ Full body

STRENGTH

EXERCISE	SETS	REPS	WEIGHT

CARDIO

	TIME	DISTANCE	INTENSITY

REST DAY

MY DAY

FOOD JOURNAL

DATE: 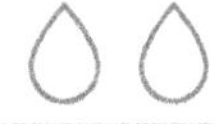 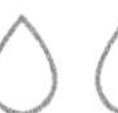 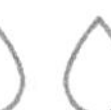

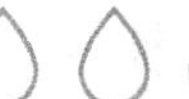 M T W T F S S

Breakfast

PROTEIN | FATS | CARBS | CALORIES

Lunch

PROTEIN | FATS | CARBS | CALORIES

Dinner

PROTEIN | FATS | CARBS | CALORIES

Snacks

PROTEIN | FATS | CARBS | CALORIES

WATER

SLEEP (HRS)

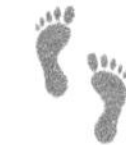

DAILY STEPS

FOCUS

☐ Legs   ☐ Arms   ☐ Abs   ☐ Full body

STRENGTH

EXERCISE	SETS	REPS	WEIGHT

CARDIO

	TIME	DISTANCE	INTENSITY

REST DAY

MY DAY

DATE: /   /   M T W T F S S

FOOD JOURNAL

Breakfast

PROTEIN	FATS	CARBS	CALORIES

Lunch

PROTEIN	FATS	CARBS	CALORIES

Dinner

PROTEIN	FATS	CARBS	CALORIES

Snacks

PROTEIN	FATS	CARBS	CALORIES

WATER

○ ○ ○ ○ ○ ○ ○ ○

SLEEP (HRS)

DAILY STEPS

FOCUS

☐ Legs   ☐ Arms   ☐ Abs   ☐ Full body

STRENGTH

EXERCISE	SETS	REPS	WEIGHT

CARDIO

	TIME	DISTANCE	INTENSITY

REST DAY

MY DAY

FOOD JOURNAL

Breakfast

PROTEIN	FATS	CARBS	CALORIES

Lunch

PROTEIN	FATS	CARBS	CALORIES

Dinner

PROTEIN	FATS	CARBS	CALORIES

Snacks

PROTEIN	FATS	CARBS	CALORIES

DATE:

M T W T F S S

WATER

SLEEP (HRS)

DAILY STEPS

FOCUS

☐ Legs ☐ Arms ☐ Abs ☐ Full body

STRENGTH

EXERCISE	SETS	REPS	WEIGHT

CARDIO

	TIME	DISTANCE	INTENSITY

REST DAY

MY DAY

DATE: / /   M T W T F S S

FOOD JOURNAL

Breakfast

PROTEIN	FATS	CARBS	CALORIES

Lunch

PROTEIN	FATS	CARBS	CALORIES

Dinner

PROTEIN	FATS	CARBS	CALORIES

Snacks

PROTEIN	FATS	CARBS	CALORIES

WATER

◇ ◇ ◇ ◇ ◇ ◇ ◇ ◇

SLEEP (HRS)

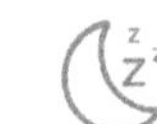

DAILY STEPS

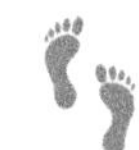

FOCUS

☐ Legs   ☐ Arms   ☐ Abs   ☐ Full body

STRENGTH

EXERCISE	SETS	REPS	WEIGHT

CARDIO

	TIME	DISTANCE	INTENSITY

REST DAY

MY DAY

DATE: ___/___/___   M T W T F S S

FOOD JOURNAL

Breakfast

PROTEIN	FATS	CARBS	CALORIES

Lunch

PROTEIN	FATS	CARBS	CALORIES

Dinner

PROTEIN	FATS	CARBS	CALORIES

Snacks

PROTEIN	FATS	CARBS	CALORIES

WATER

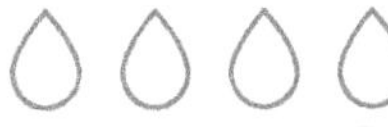 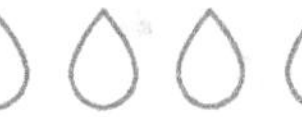 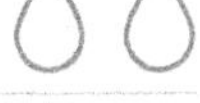

SLEEP (HRS)

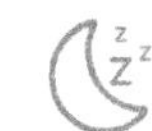

DAILY STEPS

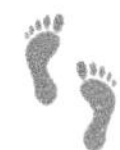

FOCUS

☐ Legs   ☐ Arms   ☐ Abs   ☐ Full body

STRENGTH

EXERCISE	SETS	REPS	WEIGHT

CARDIO

	TIME	DISTANCE	INTENSITY

REST DAY

MY DAY

DATE: / /

M T W T F S S

FOOD JOURNAL

Breakfast

PROTEIN	FATS	CARBS	CALORIES

Lunch

PROTEIN	FATS	CARBS	CALORIES

Dinner

PROTEIN	FATS	CARBS	CALORIES

Snacks

PROTEIN	FATS	CARBS	CALORIES

WATER

SLEEP (HRS)

DAILY STEPS

FOCUS

☐ Legs ☐ Arms ☐ Abs ☐ Full body

STRENGTH

EXERCISE		SETS	REPS	WEIGHT

CARDIO

	TIME	DISTANCE	INTENSITY

REST DAY

MY DAY

DATE: / /   M T W T F S S

FOOD JOURNAL

Breakfast

PROTEIN	FATS	CARBS	CALORIES

Lunch

PROTEIN	FATS	CARBS	CALORIES

Dinner

PROTEIN	FATS	CARBS	CALORIES

Snacks

PROTEIN	FATS	CARBS	CALORIES

WATER

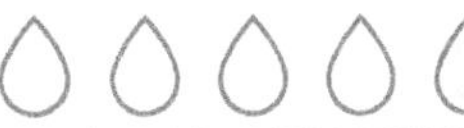

SLEEP (HRS)

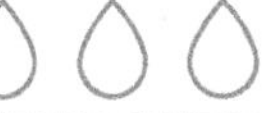

DAILY STEPS

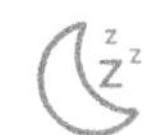

FOCUS

☐ Legs   ☐ Arms   ☐ Abs   ☐ Full body

STRENGTH

EXERCISE	SETS	REPS	WEIGHT

CARDIO

	TIME	DISTANCE	INTENSITY

REST DAY

MY DAY

FOOD JOURNAL

DATE: ___________   M T W T F S S

Breakfast

PROTEIN	FATS	CARBS	CALORIES

Lunch

PROTEIN	FATS	CARBS	CALORIES

Dinner

PROTEIN	FATS	CARBS	CALORIES

Snacks

PROTEIN	FATS	CARBS	CALORIES

WATER

◯ ◯ ◯ ◯ ◯ ◯ ◯ ◯

SLEEP (HRS)

DAILY STEPS

FOCUS

☐ Legs   ☐ Arms   ☐ Abs   ☐ Full body

STRENGTH

EXERCISE	SETS	REPS	WEIGHT

CARDIO

	TIME	DISTANCE	INTENSITY

REST DAY

MY DAY

DATE: / /

M T W T F S S

FOOD JOURNAL

Breakfast

PROTEIN	FATS	CARBS	CALORIES

Lunch

PROTEIN	FATS	CARBS	CALORIES

Dinner

PROTEIN	FATS	CARBS	CALORIES

Snacks

PROTEIN	FATS	CARBS	CALORIES

WATER ◇ ◇ ◇ ◇ ◇ ◇ ◇ ◇

SLEEP (HRS)

DAILY STEPS

FOCUS

☐ Legs ☐ Arms ☐ Abs ☐ Full body

STRENGTH

EXERCISE	SETS	REPS	WEIGHT

CARDIO

	TIME	DISTANCE	INTENSITY

REST DAY

MY DAY

DATE: /   /   M T W T F S S

FOOD JOURNAL

Breakfast

PROTEIN	FATS	CARBS	CALORIES

Lunch

PROTEIN	FATS	CARBS	CALORIES

Dinner

PROTEIN	FATS	CARBS	CALORIES

Snacks

PROTEIN	FATS	CARBS	CALORIES

WATER

SLEEP (HRS)

DAILY STEPS

FOCUS

☐ Legs ☐ Arms ☐ Abs ☐ Full body

STRENGTH

EXERCISE	SETS	REPS	WEIGHT

CARDIO

	TIME	DISTANCE	INTENSITY

REST DAY

MY DAY

DATE: ___________   M T W T F S S

FOOD JOURNAL

Breakfast

PROTEIN	FATS	CARBS	CALORIES

Lunch

PROTEIN	FATS	CARBS	CALORIES

Dinner

PROTEIN	FATS	CARBS	CALORIES

Snacks

PROTEIN	FATS	CARBS	CALORIES

WATER

〇 〇 〇 〇 〇 〇 〇 〇

SLEEP (HRS)

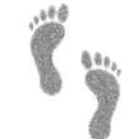

DAILY STEPS

FOCUS

☐ Legs ☐ Arms ☐ Abs ☐ Full body

STRENGTH

EXERCISE	SETS	REPS	WEIGHT

CARDIO

	TIME	DISTANCE	INTENSITY

REST DAY

MY DAY

DATE: / /   M T W T F S S

FOOD JOURNAL

Breakfast

PROTEIN	FATS	CARBS	CALORIES

Lunch

PROTEIN	FATS	CARBS	CALORIES

Dinner

PROTEIN	FATS	CARBS	CALORIES

Snacks

PROTEIN	FATS	CARBS	CALORIES

WATER ◇ ◇ ◇ ◇ ◇ ◇ ◇ ◇

SLEEP (HRS)

DAILY STEPS

FOCUS

☐ Legs   ☐ Arms   ☐ Abs   ☐ Full body

STRENGTH

EXERCISE	SETS	REPS	WEIGHT

CARDIO

	TIME	DISTANCE	INTENSITY

REST DAY

MY DAY

FOOD JOURNAL

DATE: / /

M T W T F S S

Breakfast

PROTEIN	FATS	CARBS	CALORIES

Lunch

PROTEIN	FATS	CARBS	CALORIES

Dinner

PROTEIN	FATS	CARBS	CALORIES

Snacks

PROTEIN	FATS	CARBS	CALORIES

WATER

SLEEP (HRS)

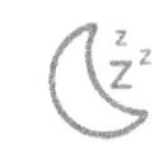

DAILY STEPS

FOCUS

☐ Legs   ☐ Arms   ☐ Abs   ☐ Full body

STRENGTH

EXERCISE	SETS	REPS	WEIGHT

CARDIO

	TIME	DISTANCE	INTENSITY

REST DAY

MY DAY

FOOD JOURNAL

Breakfast

PROTEIN   FATS   CARBS   CALORIES

Lunch

PROTEIN   FATS   CARBS   CALORIES

Dinner

PROTEIN   FATS   CARBS   CALORIES

Snacks

PROTEIN   FATS   CARBS   CALORIES

DATE: M T W T F S S

WATER

⬭ ⬭ ⬭ ⬭ ⬭ ⬭ ⬭ ⬭

SLEEP (HRS)

DAILY STEPS

FOCUS

☐ Legs   ☐ Arms   ☐ Abs   ☐ Full body

STRENGTH

EXERCISE	SETS	REPS	WEIGHT

CARDIO

	TIME	DISTANCE	INTENSITY

REST DAY

MY DAY

DATE: /   /   M T W T F S S

FOOD JOURNAL

Breakfast

PROTEIN	FATS	CARBS	CALORIES

Lunch

PROTEIN	FATS	CARBS	CALORIES

Dinner

PROTEIN	FATS	CARBS	CALORIES

Snacks

PROTEIN	FATS	CARBS	CALORIES

WATER

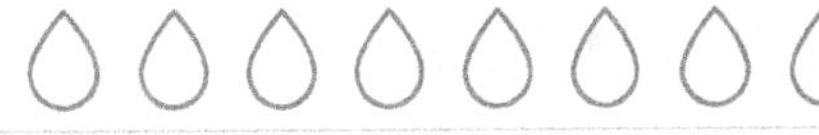

SLEEP (HRS)

DAILY STEPS

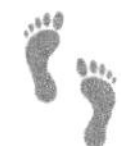

FOCUS

☐ Legs ☐ Arms ☐ Abs ☐ Full body

STRENGTH

EXERCISE	SETS	REPS	WEIGHT

CARDIO

	TIME	DISTANCE	INTENSITY

REST DAY

MY DAY

DATE: / /   M T W T F S S

FOOD JOURNAL

Breakfast

PROTEIN	FATS	CARBS	CALORIES

Lunch

PROTEIN	FATS	CARBS	CALORIES

Dinner

PROTEIN	FATS	CARBS	CALORIES

Snacks

PROTEIN	FATS	CARBS	CALORIES

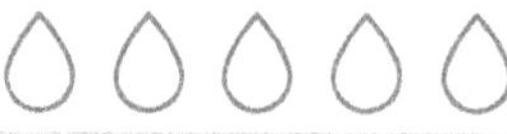

WATER ⬡⬡⬡⬡⬡⬡⬡⬡

SLEEP (HRS)

DAILY STEPS 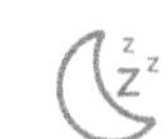

FOCUS

☐ Legs   ☐ Arms   ☐ Abs   ☐ Full body

STRENGTH

EXERCISE	SETS	REPS	WEIGHT

CARDIO

	TIME	DISTANCE	INTENSITY

REST DAY

MY NOTES

MY NOTES

MY NOTES

MY NOTES